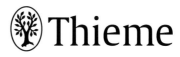

Update: Muscle injuries after 45 years of professional sports care

Diagnosis and therapy of neurogenic muscle hardening, muscle strain, muscle fiber tear and muscle bundle tear

Dr. med. Hans-Wilhelm Müller-Wohlfahrt

in collaboration with Dr. med. Sebastian Torka and Kilian Müller-Wohlfahrt

13 figures

Georg Thieme Verlag
Stuttgart · New York

Address

Dr. med. Hans-Wilhelm Müller-Wohlfahrt
Dienerstraße 12
Alter Hof
80331 München
Germany
info@mw-oc.de

*Bibliographic information published
by the Deutsche Nationalbibliothek*

The Deutsche Nationalbibliothek lists this
publication in the Deutsche Nationalbibliografie;
detailed bibliographic data is available in the
Internet at http://dnb.d-nb.de.

The printing of this booklet was made possible by
the friendly support of Heel GmbH, Baden-Baden,
Germany.

Medical writers:
Dr. med. Sebastian Torka, München
Kilian Müller-Wohlfahrt, München

© 2021. Thieme. All rights reserved.
Georg Thieme Verlag KG
Rüdigerstraße 14, 70469 Stuttgart, Germany
www.thieme.de

Printed in Germany

Coverdesign: © Thieme
Image source cover:
Soccer player: © luchioly/stock.adobe.com
Two soccer players: © Maxisport/stock.adobe.com
Typesetting: Ziegler + Müller, Kirchentellinsfurt
Print and Bookbinding:
Westermann Druck Zwickau GmbH, Zwickau

ISBN   978-3-13-244370-9

Contents

Acknowledgements

Many thanks for the textual revision and co-design by Hannes Degenhardt on behalf of the Sports Orthopaedics Department of the Technical University Hospital rechts der Isar.

Special thanks are also due to Imke Bergmann, my right hand for many years.

1 Introduction

One of the most difficult tasks in sports medicine is, in my opinion, to diagnose muscle injuries exactly and to devise the appropriate therapy and training protocol (Fig. 1).

Medical history, symptoms, palpation of muscle injuries, functional tests and identification of the underlying cause are crucial to initiate the right treatment steps at the right time.

Care must be taken not to take any risks and to avoid a recurrence, but also to ensure that no time is lost and that the injured person is returned to full activity as soon as possible.

Based on the diagnosis, the duration of treatment can be predicted quite accurately. This is also important for the injured person because it gives him or her an insight and a target to work towards.

In addition to the medical history, daily palpation is of elementary importance, as it is the only way – depending on the current findings – to manage the rehabilitation responsibly and to increase the training load depending on the palpatory findings. It should not mean: "*Just try it, maybe it will work.*" There is no possibility of "trial and error".

Under no circumstances may the management be directed by symptoms, as the pain will already ease before the healing process is complete. Too early loading means a significantly increased risk of re-injury.

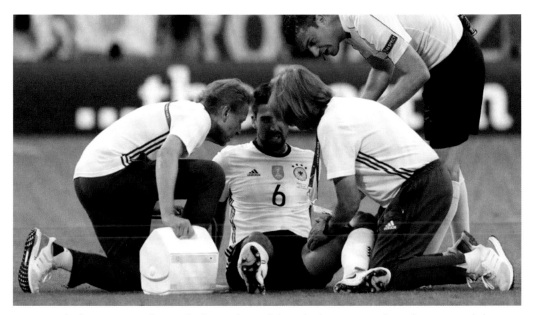

Fig. 1 Medical examination of Sami Khedira on the pitch (2016): The important factor here is a quick diagnosis and a decision as to whether it is possible to continue playing.

2 Classification

If in my early days as a sports physician in the 1970 s, muscle injuries were differentiated purely quantitatively, we were already able to make a qualitative differentiation in the 1980 s and develop the following classification (Table 1) [1].

The essential point is that for the first time we separated and listed the structural from the functional (non-structural) muscle injuries individually. This had a significant impact on the types of therapy and the duration of treatment.

Our Munich Classification was declared years ago as the basis for the UEFA's injury studies in the Champions League clubs.

UEFA definition of injury: An injury is when the athlete stops the match or training because of pain.

The following chapters describe this in detail. I think this is important because at the end of this article I would like to compare the theoretical and impractical magnetic resonance imaging (MRI) diagnostics with clinical diagnostics.

I very much regret that magnetic resonance diagnostics are increasingly being used at the cost of clinical examination.

Table 1 Munich Consensus Classification for the classification of muscle injuries according to Müller-Wohlfahrt [1].

A. Indirect muscle injuries	functional (= not structural)	Type 1: due to overload	Type 1A: fatigue-related muscle hardening
			Type 1B: muscle soreness = DOMS
		Type 2: neuromuscular	Type 2A: neurogenic muscle hardening
			Type 2B: muscle strain
	structural	Type 3: partial rupture	Type 3A: muscle fiber rupture
			Type 3B: muscle bundle rupture
		Type 4: (sub-)total rupture	subtotal/total muscle rupture, tendinous avulsion
B. Direct muscle injuries		contusion	
		laceration	

Table **2**   Radiological classification of muscle injuries, British Athletic Muscle Injury Classification [2, 3].

Grade	Extent of edema	Site	Architectural disruption
0	Nil	Nil	Nil
1: small tear	< 10 % CSA < 5 cm long	a. myofascial b. MTJ	< 1-cm gap < 1-cm gap
2: moderate tear	10–50 % CSA 5–15 cm long	a. myofascial b. MTJ c. tendon < 50 % CSA	a. 1- to 5-cm gap b. 1- to 5-cm gap c. no redundancy, no gap
3: extensive tear	> 50 % CSA > 15 cm long	a. myofascial b. MTJ c. tendon > 50 % CSA	a. > 5-cm gap b. > 5-cm gap c. tendon redundancy
4: complete tear			complete muscle tear complete tendon tear with retraction

CSA = cross-sectional area, MTJ = muscle-tendon junction

This trend is a source of great concern to me because I simply consider MRI examinations unsuitable due to frequent misdiagnosis (of muscle injuries), this leads many colleagues on the wrong track. MRI images are often misinterpreted and overrated and too much trust is placed in MRI.

Therefore, I also consider an MRI-based classification to be wrong and unsuitable such as the frequently used radiological classification of Dimmick and Linklater (Table **2**) [2]).

3 Medical history

The medical history is an elementary component of a detailed diagnosis (Fig. 2). We are often led on the right track simply by asking specific questions when taking the medical history:

1. How many hours/days have passed since the injury?
2. What did the athlete notice? How did he experience the injury?
3. Did he feel pain? Was the pain sharp or blunt?
4. Was it a cramp-like pain that developed over several steps or was it of sudden onset?
5. Did he notice painful traction?
6. Was the pain localized or did the pain affect the muscle in its entire length?
7. Was there any previous evidence of muscle fatigue?
8. Did the injured muscle stretch well previously during warm-up or did it take longer than usual?
9. Was the muscle warmed up and stretched specifically for the sport?
10. Did the legs feel heavy before the injury?
11. Was the training on unfamiliar surfaces (e.g. hard court, frozen floor)? The muscle tone can be increased through joint-specific proprioception!
12. Were the shoes changed? Have the insoles been forgotten?
13. Were there any new training contents to which a trained and highly sensitive muscle reacts more often with an injury?
14. Was there a change of coach or club?
15. How high was the training load in the last days?
16. How many matches took place in which period?
17. Were the training breaks sufficient?
18. Was there previously an injury to muscles or tendons in the area of the movement chain?
19. Was there a feeling of restricted movement or even pain in the area of the adjacent joints?
20. Has the spine caused problems?
21. Was there an infection?
22. Were the laboratory values normal, e.g. uric acid, whose value should in any case be below 6 mg/dl?
23. In this context one more important observation: Did the athlete fall to the ground after the injury (such as Tyson Gay, Fig. 3) or could he still walk slowly and try to continue playing?

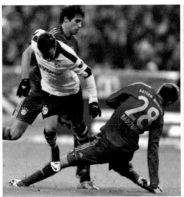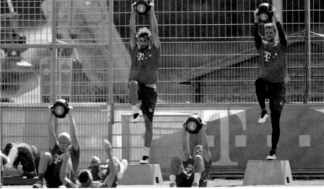

Fig. 2 Anamnesis for a precise evaluation of the injury mechanism, the symptoms before and after the injury and other medical and sports-related factors.

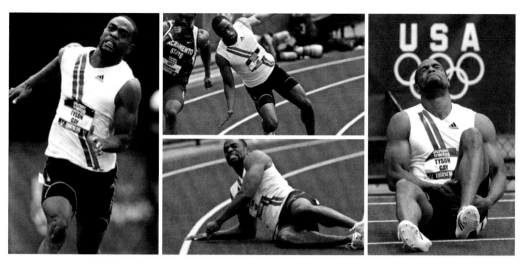

Fig. **3**   Tyson Gay suffers a rupture of the left hamstring muscle bundle during the 200-meter sprint (U. S. athletics championship, quarter-final, 2008) and falls to the ground. Afterward, he will be treated in our practice.

3.1   Symptoms of the respective injuries

3.1.1   Symptoms of neurogenic muscle hardening (2A)

Neurogenic muscle hardening (2A) is not always easy to distinguish from muscle strain. However, a characteristic feature is that the increased muscle tension extends over the entire length of a muscle strand, sometimes even a muscle group. Depending on the cause, you may experience a pulling sensation, an increasing feeling of tension and finally real pain.

The muscle is felt as rigid, inelastic and shortened, e.g. during a soccer match. The athlete no longer feels secure and therefore changes his position to avoid long sprints in quick succession. He remains reserved in his way of playing. The danger of a torn muscle fiber during the sprint is particularly high in this phase and the athlete is aware of this. This can lead to the athlete being replaced. The explanation is then: *"Coach, the muscle has blocked"*, which hits the core of the complaints very well.

According to our experience, neurogenic muscle hardening is probably the most common muscle injury of all, due to which an athlete has to stop his training or match.

3.1.2   Symptoms of muscle strain (2B)

In the case of muscle strain (2B), the cramp-like pain is usually not acute, so that the injured person often still believes that he or she can continue playing. At a slow pace, this may be possible at the beginning of a strain. At higher intensity, however, the pain increases rapidly, i.e. the tone continues to increase unphysiologically and the athlete is slowed down by a presumably hypoxemic pain.

The pain only affects a limited muscle segment. The athlete feels the need to stretch the muscle but soon realizes that this does not solve the problem.

3.1.3 Symptoms of a muscle fiber rupture (3A)

In the case of a muscle fiber rupture (3A) – we speak of a rupture of a so-called flesh fiber, i.e. a secondary bundle up to 5 mm thick (surrounded by the perimysium externum) – the injured person usually feels a sharp, one could say needle-stick-like, pain. Less frequently, the injury is perceived as a sharp burning sensation. The athlete immediately adopts a compensatory posture or gait. He knows that it is not possible to continue playing because he immediately realizes that the injury would get worse.

3.1.4 Symptoms of a muscle bundle rupture (3B)

In the case of a muscle bundle rupture (3B), the athlete suffers a dull, knife-like pain and falls to the ground. The fall is due to a protective reflex to prevent further damage. Exceptions are extremely rare here. He no longer dares to get up or walk without help. He knows that he has been seriously injured.

3.1.5 Symptoms of a partial tear or muscle tear (4)

In the case of a partial tear (4) or muscle tear (4), the pain is so severe that the injured person no longer makes any attempt to stand up or walk.

4   Examination

It must be admitted that the examination of the skeletal muscles requires some experience and good empathy. Intuitive talent is also beneficial.

At the beginning of the palpation, which has to be performed without time pressure and in a calm environment, the attention, the concentration increases – I get familiar with the anatomical conditions.

Palpation of muscle injuries in the lower extremity is facilitated by the fact that we can examine against an abutment (femur, tibia, fibula) and the muscle is not able to move. Therefore, the examination of the abdominal muscles is much more difficult.

Based on the patient's specific injury, medical history and my evaluation, I practically pre-program myself in this phase and remember all the impressions and sensations that I associate, for ex-

ample, with a torn or strained muscle fiber. I must therefore know what I am looking for during palpation. In the process of my work as a sports medicine specialist, I have examined countless muscle injuries and stored them in my memory, so that I have a clear idea of every possible injury.

I assign the impressions gained during palpation to existing memory contents, so-called engrams, in order to come to a diagnosis.

In addition, passive and active functional diagnostics in the entire physiological range of motion are recommended as part of the diagnostic process.

Prior to the examination, the patient is positioned to ensure that the muscles to be examined are relaxed, and a second examination session is performed in a slightly tensioned state (Fig. 4 and Fig. 5).

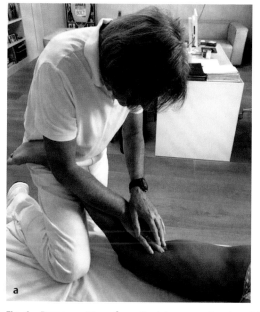 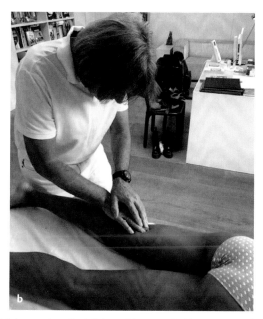

Fig. 4   Prone position of a patient to assess the dorsal thigh muscles of a left leg with an angled knee joint and relaxed muscles (**a**) and with a stretched knee joint and slightly tensed muscles (**b**).

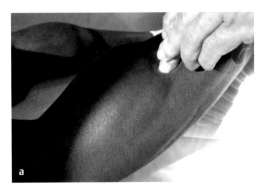 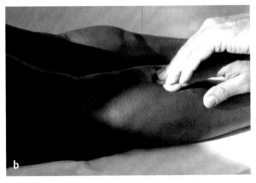

Fig. **5**   Palpation of a left lower leg, sliding with slight pressure with the fingertip with relaxed (**a**) and slightly tensed (**b**) muscles while looking for a hypertonic muscle bundle.

At first, I get a differentiated impression of the muscle tone of the non-injured side in order to get to know the physiological state of tension of the individual athlete. Then I repeatedly glide my hand over a large area of the injured region to gain impressions of the skin, subcutaneous tissue, fascia and, to a certain extent, the muscles. I also feel the temperature and then search for a shortened muscle strand or muscle bundle via palpation, which has a higher tone than the surrounding muscles. Experience shows that this muscle bundle contains the injury of whichever kind.

This is done with medium pressure and by moving the skin so that I slide my fingertip over the muscle (Fig. **5**). I then try to locate the injury in this muscle bundle – usually with my eyes closed – by repeated sliding palpation from proximal to distal and back or even across the direction of the fibers. Simply pressing down is not enough.

In order to complete the palpation, an ultrasound examination can be useful, although it cannot replace the palpation. The quality of the equipment and the experience of the examiner are certainly the limiting factors here. However, it provides important visual information about the injury and the healing process.

Magnetic resonance imaging is being used more and more. In my opinion, however, it is not suitable for providing an exact image in the case of minor injuries, such as strained muscles, neurogenic hardening or torn muscle fibers. All too often it exaggerates the injury. I also cannot accept the MRI-based grading of injury severity from 1 to 3, as it is made dependent on the extent of the hematoma or edema.

For example, the same injury is considered less severe after optimal first aid (compression and ice water) than if no first aid is given.

Functional muscle injuries are not recorded at all.

4.1   The importance of palpation in my personal career at FC Bayern Munich

In the 1976/77 season I was responsible for the care of the licensed players of FC Bayern Munich (Fig. **6**). The demands on me were very high right from the start. The club had won the European Cup for the 3rd time and it was simply expected that I could make the right diagnosis already in the arena and initiate the best possible therapy.

I was on my own, diagnostic tools in the stadiums such as ultrasound equipment were not available at that time.

I had no other choice but to practice and train myself, especially in the palpation of injuries, because I could prepare myself for the fact that promptly after an injury the question was asked by the coach or even the manager: "*What is wrong with the player? When can he play again?*" And this is still considered the standard today. For understandable reasons, mistakes are unacceptable.

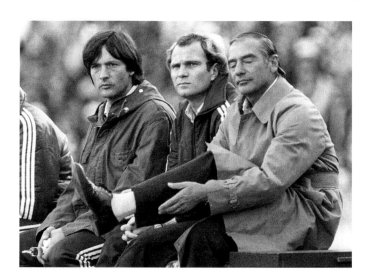

Fig. **6** The coach bench of FC Bayern Munich (1978); from left to right: Dr. med. Hans-Wilhelm Müller-Wohlfahrt, Ulrich Hoeneß, Pál Csernai.

4.2 Results of the examination

In the following, I will try to describe the qualities of the individual muscle lesions as precisely as possible.

4.2.1 Examination findings of neurogenic muscle hardening (2A)

The affected muscle bundle is hypertonic in its entire extension and also shows an edematous seam between muscle and fascia over its entire length, which can be visualized on ultrasound examination and MRI (Fig. **7**). This is usually 1–2 mm thick and gives the impression of a fluid accumulation that feels strangely "soapy". I was almost always able to make this tactile finding in cases of neurogenic muscle hardening, without knowing the reason.

Since the fluid cushion to be palpated is pure lymphatic congestion, the tactile findings can be explained by the composition of the lymph fluid. This is due to the glucosaminoglycans and proteoglycans contained in the lymph fluid, which bind water and thus give the lymph fluid a "soapy" consistency.

On palpation, the muscle reacts with tenderness under pressure. Even the skin over the injury is sometimes sensitive or painful to touch. During stretching, the pulling effect is intensified.

Muscle hardening as a result of **fatigue** must be clearly distinguished from the neurogenic type. It does not show edema – e.g. after high training load. We call the hardening "dry". The athlete usually notices it the next day.

4.2.1.1 Genesis of neurogenic muscle hardening

The cause of increased muscle tension is due to a pathological innervation by the supplying motor nerve, which experiences a mechanical stimulus in the area of the spinal column or the sacroiliac joint (entrapment) and responds by overregulating the muscle (increased pulse rate). The accompanying vegetative nerve fibers cause – according to my hypothesis – a dysregulation in the lymph vessel system and usually lead to a lymph stasis, which can be felt like a fluid seam.

In cases of severe misinnervation, lymphatic stasis can also be found outside the fascia and can then – locally and/or over a long distance – assume considerably larger dimensions and present itself as a clearly visible swelling, as we sometimes see in the adductor region.

Since the 1980s, I have repeatedly lectured and written about the phenomenon of "lymph stasis in neurogenic muscle hardening".

At that time, there were no scientific studies or publications on the topic of "innervation of lymph vessels". Even today, very little is known about it.

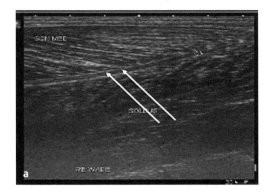

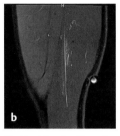
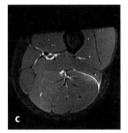

Fig. **7**   Visualization of an edema seam along the muscle fascia in neurogenic muscle hardening in ultrasound examination (**a**; white arrows) and MRI imaging in sagittal (**b**) and axial planes (**c**).

In this regard, I have held various discussions with renowned specialists in this field. In the following, I will present the contents of an expert discussion with Prof. Dr. Dr. med. Michael Schünke (former director of the anatomical institute of the University of Kiel):

At least the lymph collectors, which connect to the initial lymph vessels (capillaries), have a smooth muscular media in the valve-free collector segment, which is capable of rhythmical successive contraction waves and thus transports the lymph. Smooth musculature is always visceral-efferently innervated, whereby the switchover from the 1st to the 2nd sympathetic neuron is localized in the sympathetic trunk ganglion. The postganglionic neuron then finds its way to the vessels of the lower extremity via the corresponding ramus ventralis, the plexus lumbosacralis and further along the peripheral nerves (e.g. femoral nerve).

This means that the **blood vessels (certain) and also the lymph vessels (very likely) are sympathetically innervated**. *If there is a subliminal irritation of the motor nerves, the vegetative fibers are usually also affected.*

While the motor fibers are protected by a thick myelin sheath against the effect of slight pressure, the sheathless fibers of the sympathetic nervous system have little structural protection. As a result of this, in the event of impingement, they can no longer fulfill their function. This results in vasodilatation of the blood vessels and – it is assumed – of the lymph vessels.

Both together could therefore result in a localized accumulation of lymph fluid due to dysregulation. Presumably, lymphatic vessels with contractile wall sections are only found after passing through the muscle fascia. This means: Inside the muscle (intramuscular = inside the fascia) the transport of lymph fluid is regulated exclusively via the so-called initial lymph vessels (lymph capillaries).

4.2.2   Examination findings of muscle strain (2B)

The muscle strain is usually located in the area of the muscle belly and can be felt as a spindle-shaped thickening in an extension of about 15–20 cm. It is moderately painful under pressure and tolerates – in contrast to the structural and neurogenic injuries – a slight stretching without counter-reaction. The muscle tone is increased in the extension of the muscle strain – i.e. a limited section of the injured muscle strand. The injured muscle shows no edema, no hematoma is found. This injury cannot be diagnosed based on MRI examination.

4.2.2.1 Genesis of muscle strain

Muscle strain is a functional, neuromuscular, rather than a structural injury. In my opinion, this is due to a dysregulation by the muscle spindles, which are responsible for measuring the length of the respective muscles and run parallel to the striated muscles.

Similar to the Golgi tendon organ (tension receptor of the tendon), the muscle spindle belongs to the proprioceptors and is therefore sensitive to stimuli that are generated in its locomotor system. The interaction of agonists and antagonists is very complex in movement sequences and this dynamic process must be constantly coordinated by the respective feedback of the proprioceptors.

Furthermore, it is known that the impulse frequency of the muscle spindles and the action potential frequency of the Ia afferents is proportional to the length of the muscle and the speed at which a change in length occurs.

If there is a rapid change in muscle length during sport-specific load peaks and the muscle spindles are not prepared, one could say not adjusted accordingly, they react with increased impulse frequencies via the afferent nerves to the transition zone at the spinal cord. Here they cause a malfunction in the functional units with dysregulation of the agonists and antagonists.

On the one hand, an increased action potential is then fired from the anterior horn of the spinal cord via the α motor neuron back to the muscle (to the motor endplate of the agonist), where it causes an increased contraction of the innervated muscle fibers.

On the other hand, Ia interneurons are strongly activated. Normally, these cause a reciprocal inhibition of the antagonists via the α motor neurons. However, during the genesis of muscle strain, the inhibitory effect on the antagonists is missing.

Crucial for this are the Renshaw cells and Ia interneurons, whose function it is to regulate the strength of the inhibition. In the case of excitation (overstimulation) of Renshaw cells and Ia interneurons from the muscle spindles, they will degenerate into dysfunction (malfunction) and cause a failure of reciprocal inhibition.

For example, after a quantitatively and qualitatively insufficient warm-up and stretching (dynamic) before training or competition, suddenly occurring rapid strength movements or a rapid change of rhythm can lead to cramp-like muscle problems, which are initially perceived as a sensation of discomfort (e.g. a feeling of cold).

When the load is continued and intensified, for example with even faster running, they are felt more intensely and finally as pain.

If the training or competition is continued, the activity of the α motor neurons leading to the agonist increases continuously and at the same time

the tone of the muscle fibers supplied by them increases, while the antagonists are not inhibited accordingly.

This makes the spindle-shaped extension of the strain understandable.

The agonist now works against the resistance of the antagonist and, if the athletic activity is continued and the tone of the muscle increases continuously, the agonist reaches a painful, cramp-like state that requires a cessation of the activity. The muscle pain cannot be classified as acute because it increases gradually during exercise. At least that is my clinical experience and theoretical hypothesis.

There is little scientific knowledge or literature on the pathophysiological dysregulation of muscle tone as a result of a muscle spindle dysfunction. A pressure effect on the muscle spindle membrane in one way or another is hypothesized to be the cause of this, following a literature search and expert discussion with Prof. Dr. Michael Dimitriou (Professor at the Department of Integrative Medical Biology [IMB], Sweden) and Prof. Dr. med. Timm Filler (Section Head of Clinical Anatomy, University of Düsseldorf) [4].

Note: The function of the muscle spindles is temperature-dependent. Therefore, to prevent muscle strain, it is essential to condition the muscle spindles to bring about an even activity level and to increase the reactivity by a sport-specific, time-consuming warm-up. Once the highest possible muscle elasticity has been achieved as a result of the warm-up and dynamic stretching, hypersensitivity to stretching stimuli is reduced, thus raising the threshold for incipient reflex mechanisms. This minimizes the risk of muscle spindle dysregulation resulting in muscle strain.

4.2.3 Examination findings of the muscle fiber rupture (3A)

Here, generally large fiber interruptions in a hypertonic muscle strand, which lie in the millimeter range (up to about 5 mm), are noticeable and can be felt with the fingertip. In the first few minutes, the gap is filled with only a minimal amount of blood, but in the following minutes more and more blood accumulates here. The injury is then difficult to palpate since the fascia is usually uninjured, i.e. it is an intramuscular injury. The torn muscle fiber is very painful under pressure.

If, in addition, extensive edema is present along the injured muscle strand, it can be assumed that a neurogenic malfunction of the muscle and the lymph vessel system already existed before the injury and that the muscle was consequently prone to injury.

In the hours following the injury, an inflammatory reaction lasting several days (approx. five days) develops with swelling of the injured region. The parts of the affected muscle bundle immediately proximal and distal to the torn muscle fiber, as well as directly adjacent muscle bundles, often assume a much higher tone after the injury.

I consider this to be a natural response to protect the injured muscle structures. This finding can only be established by palpation. No imaging technique is capable to achieve this. Equally important is the fact that this protective tension only decreases after the injury has completely healed. Therefore, this symptom forms the basis for the decision to reintegrate into training.

4.2.4   Examination of muscle bundle tear (3B)

This injury is most likely to be found in the muscle-tendon transition area, is extremely painful due to pressure and movement, and can usually be clearly defined as a gap measuring more than 5 mm at the fingertips, when palpation is performed with almost pressure-free sliding. The fascia surrounding the muscle bundle is also injured. As a rule, there is extensive bleeding, i.e. an intermuscular hematoma which finds its way into the subcutaneous tissue and becomes externally visible.

5 Therapy of muscle injuries

The sports physiotherapist and doctor treat the patient collaboratively and discuss the findings and the appropriate therapeutic approach daily in order to achieve the fastest possible healing.

In principle, the regeneration and new formation of muscle fibers takes about 10 to 14 days in the case of torn muscle fibers and the new formation of muscle fibers and collagen fibers takes about 6 weeks in the case of torn muscle bundles. It is crucial that the healing process begins in the first minute. Since the development of a hematoma in muscle injuries leads to an impairment of healing, one of the therapeutic goals is to minimize bleeding.

The following principle applies to all muscle injuries mentioned above:
1. No strength training until the injury is completely healed!
2. Cortisone or painkillers are not used – also not to suppress symptoms.

In summary, the therapy of muscle injuries is clearly shown in Table **3**.

Table **3**   Therapy and duration of downtime for muscle injuries; classification according to Müller-Wohlfahrt.

Muscle Injury – type (classification according to Müller-Wohlfahrt)	Physical measures	Infiltration therapy	Duration of absence
Neurogenic muscle hardening (2A)	Detonising electrical therapy (muscle) manual therapy lumbar spine	Infiltration therapy (muscle) (Meaverin® 1.0%, Actovegin® and Traumeel®) comprehensive spinal physiotherapy (usually several segments)	Running training from day 1 post trauma at low-stress level, return to full capacity after 2–3 days
Muscle strain (2B)	Hot-ice, muscle release, strain-counterstrain, spray and stretch	Infiltration therapy (muscle), possibly repetition day 2 post trauma (Meaverin® 1.0%, Actovegin®, Traumeel®)	Running training in the painless range from day 1 post trauma, full load capacity after 3–5 days
Muscle fiber rupture (3A)	Hot-ice, compression and positioning, from day 2, lymph drainage	Infiltration therapy (muscle) day 1, day 3 and day 5 (Meaverin® 1.0%, Actovegin® Traumee®l)	Running training from day 6, absence from sport 10–14 days
Muscle bundle rupture (3B)	Hot-ice, compression and positioning, from day 2 lymph drainage	Infiltration therapy (muscle) day 1, day 3 and day 5 (Meaverin® 1.0%, Actovegin® Traumeel®)	After 4 weeks start with bike ergometer training, after 5 weeks start with running training, after 6–7 weeks full load

5.1   Therapy of neurogenic muscle hardening (2A)

In neurogenic etiology, where we usually find the cause of the misinnervation in the area of the spinal cord segments to be assigned, the following procedure is followed:
1. Initially infiltration of the affected muscle strand in its entire length according to the treatment of the torn muscle fiber (see chapter 5.3).
2. To achieve fast and lasting treatment success, a comprehensive therapy of the corresponding spinal column segments is then carried out (see chapter 6).

Immediately afterwards, this often leads to a relaxation in the pain-causing muscle, which the patient experiences with relief. As general rule, running training at a low load level can be started after 1 day and the usual training program can be resumed after 2 – 3 days.

I recommend to proceed in the given order: If the spinal column is treated first, finding the hypertonic muscle strand to be treated can be difficult because of a spontaneous loss of tone. If infiltration therapy of the spine and the muscle is not carried out, there is a risk of a training interruption lasting days, sometimes weeks. Physical measures such as a light massage also do not have any effect or only a very gradual effect. The condition improves only for a short time, but after half an hour of training at the latest, the muscle returns to its old condition. The shortened muscle does not release from its tension. The muscle does not tolerate classic and strong massage techniques in this phase. They can even cause a worsening of the findings, since the nerve fibers running through the muscle, which are already irritated, may cause a further increase in tone. In this condition, the nerve fibers can be easily palpated with experienced palpation.

5.2   Therapy of muscle strain (2B)

After the first physical measures (such as hot-ice, muscle release, strain-counterstrain, spray and stretch) on the day of the injury, we recommend infiltration therapy via several needles into the injured muscle strand to achieve an isometric reduction in tone by blocking the innervation and improving the energy metabolism in the area of the injury, as in the case of muscle fiber rupture (see chapter 5.3) with Meaverin® (1.0%), Actovegin® and Traumeel®.

If necessary, this therapeutic procedure is repeated on the 2nd day after the injury. We consider running training (jogging) in the pain-free area from the 1st, at the latest 2nd day after the injury, i. e. at the earliest possible time (early functional), to be a therapeutic measure. The injured muscle as a result of a neuromuscular malfunction – I am thinking of reciprocal inhibition that has temporarily ceased to function – is trained in its function and thus returned to its accustomed performance level more quickly, usually after 3 –5 days.

Muscle hardening due to high training load, i.e. **fatigue**, on the other hand, can be loosened very well by physical applications in combination with massages.

5.3   Therapy of the muscle fiber rupture (3A)

In the case of a torn muscle fiber, the very first measure (hot-ice, compression, elevated positioning) serves to keep bleeding as low as possible. On the one hand, this is done to limit the effect of structurally damaging proteolytic enzymes to a level that is physiologically necessary for healing.

The other objective is to reduce undesired inflammatory reactions, avoid adhesions, counteract an increase in tone in the affected muscle bundle within the first few hours, and promote, accelerate and control solid healing. This is done through our infiltration therapy, which is saving a lot of time. We see no sense in a wait-and-see attitude.

Our experience shows that, for example, every minute missed during the initial treatment (in the form of a large-area pressure bandage that is re-

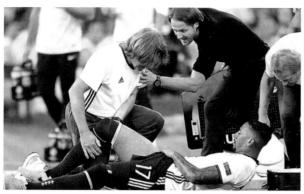
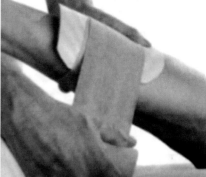

Fig. **8** Primary treatment of a muscle injury with hot-ice (right).

peatedly soaked with ice water; Fig. **8**) can mean a day's loss of time during healing. This applies up to 10 minutes. The pressure bandage may be loosened briefly after 20 minutes at the earliest and then re-applied. It should therefore be noted that post-traumatic hematoma is a kind of antagonist in the treatment for us therapists.

Infiltration therapy is performed immediately after initial treatment and on the 2nd and 4th day post trauma. It is suitable for normalizing muscle tone and thus optimizing blood supply, supporting energy and structural metabolism, keeping the inflammatory reaction low and loosening existing adhesions.

For this purpose, a mixture of Traumeel® and Actovegin® is infiltrated exactly into the center of the injury as well as proximally and distally through approx. 5–7 needles in a ratio of 1:2 (approx. 2 ml per needle). Prior to this, the needles are inserted into the muscle bundle almost painlessly with the continuous release of Meaverine® (1.0%) (Fig. **9**). In addition, zinc, magnesium, enzymes and vitamins A, C and E are prescribed per os to promote healing.

Depending on the findings during palpation, we start running at endurance running speed on the 5th/6th day after the injury (20 minutes). By increasing the running time and intensity daily, we reach the maximum load after about 10–12 days before we can start game training.

By this time, new muscle fibers have already formed after our treatments, the fiber interruption

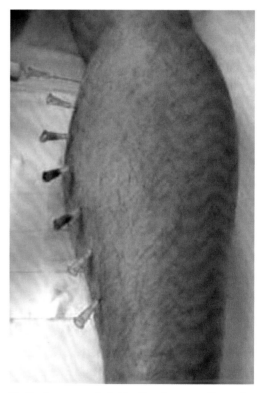

Fig. **9** Seven-needle infiltration therapy with a mixture of Traumeel® and Actovegin® of the medial gastrocnemius muscle of a right lower leg.

is closed, which was proven in a scientific study by Prof. Dr. Dr. Franz-Xaver Reichl (Ludwig-Maximilians-University of Munich) in cooperation with Prof. Dr. med. Wilhelm Bloch (Sports University of Cologne) [5]. After healing of the torn muscle fiber no scar tissue will remain.

5.4 Therapy of the muscle bundle rupture (3B)

The initial treatment, infiltration therapy as well as drug treatment (zinc, magnesium, vitamins A, C and E, enzymes) is carried out in the same way as for torn muscle fibers (3A).

Due to the severity of the injury, we recommend complete rest for 10–14 days (crutches, elevated position, relieving tape bandage) with DVT prophylaxis and accompanying lymph drainage. From the 7th day onwards, muscle massages are started proximally and distally to the injury. Furthermore, it is important to prevent adhesions. After four weeks, we start with bike ergometer training at a very low load level and depending on the palpatory findings, running training is continued after five weeks for about 10 days with increasing intensity. Following this, return to performance training commences. In contrast to a torn muscle fiber, a torn muscle bundle leaves scar tissue behind.

6 The importance of the spine in the genesis of torn muscle fibers

In the course of my many years of caring for top athletes and treating countless muscle injuries, I concluded at an early stage that about 90% of all muscle fiber/bundle tears are caused by damage or dysfunction in the spine or sacroiliac joints. This can cause nerve root irritation with the consequence that the nerve impulse output to the muscle increases, the tone of the muscle to be supplied increases and the muscle overregulates. The athlete then feels an increase in muscle tension and a decrease in elasticity. In this case, the risk of injury increases considerably.

The spinal dysfunction must also be treated if this is indicated after the examination of an athlete. Only then one can speak of complex and causal therapy of muscle injuries.

Correspondingly, I was able to determine that if the spinal column or sacroiliac joints and their disruptive factors were also treated, the healing process of the torn muscle fiber/bundle could be significantly supported.

It is therefore important to find out in which segment of the spine the source of the disorder is located.

Relevant investigations:
- Spinal and pelvic radiographs in standing position with raster to determine the real leg length difference with millimeter accuracy, which is approximately compensated.
- Functional images of the spinal column
- MRI
- CT-scan
- Scintigraphy
- EMG
- Laboratory tests (e.g. HLAB-27, uric acid, streptococcus and staphylococcus titers, zinc, magnesium, iron, copper and vitamin D_3)
- Functional investigations: If a malposition or functional abnormality indicates a:
  1. causatory intervertebral disc
  2. vertebral joint blocking
  3. inflammation in the area of joints, ligaments, muscles
  4. instability
  5. hypermobility/stiffness
  6. or pelvic misalignment, a deformity or torsion in the area of the sacrum – ileum?
- Palpatory findings for evaluation
  1. the skin, subcutaneous tissue and muscle fascia,
  2. the muscle tone (may differ segmentally),
  3. the responsiveness of tender (tendon area) and trigger points (muscle area) – they can be regarded as sensitive indicators of root irritation,
  4. the joint capsules,
  5. the ligaments,
  6. the periosteum,
  7. the irritability of the nerve root with deep finger pressure,
  8. the position of the vertebrae, sacrum, iliac bones

All relevant dysfunctions are treated simultaneously, initially with an infiltration therapy for segment relaxation, muscle tone normalization and pain relief.

Subsequently – depending on the findings – the treatment is continued with manual therapy, massages, eventually osteopathy as well as physiotherapeutic exercises to maintain mobility and improve stability.

In principle, it must be remembered that a peripheral motor nerve is composed of nerve fibers from several spinal cord segments. In spinal disorders, the mobility disorder usually affects several vertebral joints and the muscular tension of the deep paravertebral muscles – including the rotators and multifidi muscles – often extends over several spinal segments. Infiltrations (epidural, paravertebral, intracapsular) must therefore also be carried out in the area of the affected segments (usually two to three, Fig. **10**).

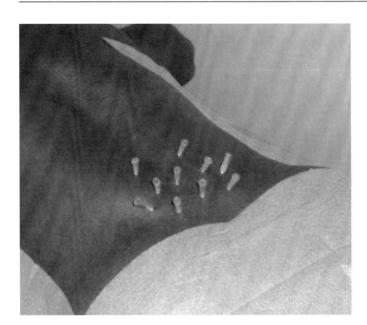

Fig. **10**   Symmetrical infiltration therapy of the spinal column with epidural, paravertebral and intracapsular infiltration.

The paravertebral infiltrations are applied symmetrically on both sides of the spine. This is to avoid or compensate for an imbalance in the affected segment, given the very high efficiency of this treatment (e.g. significant muscle relaxation).

The sacroiliac joints and the ligamentous apparatus between the spine and the pelvis (e.g. the iliolumbar ligament, which causes extremely unpleasant pain radiating along the iliac crest when irritated) are usually also treated, while the trigger and tender points are only treated in individual cases.

In this context, the sacroiliac joints lead to an unphysiological tension of the paravertebral muscles and the gluteal muscles when loaded asymmetrically. As auxiliary joints, they are unable to permanently compensate for the loss of function of the lower lumbar vertebral joints and ultimately represent an additional problem.

7 Molecular biological therapy

Note: For me as the author of this booklet there exists no conflict of interest for the drugs and active ingredients listed here. I have never received a consulting fee for their mention nor is there a contractual relationship with one of the manufacturers. They are used purely based on our conviction of their efficacy and the positive experience we have gained over decades in the treatment of muscle injuries.

7.1 Traumeel®

To clarify the mechanism of action, it has been shown that Traumeel® inhibits the secretion of the inflammatory mediators (IL-1β, TNF-α, and IL-8) up to 70 % in activated human lymphocytes [8].

Furthermore, it is known that certain herbal components of the preparation stimulate lymphocytes to synthesize and release the anti-inflammatory cytokine TGF-β and that glycoproteins from certain medicinal plants slow down the influx of inflammatory cells and their mediators. A comprehensive study of RNA sequencing showed that Traumeel® intervenes in wound healing and inflammatory processes [9].

In addition, the acidotic situation of the inflamed tissue can be buffered by the alkalizing effect of Traumeel®, thus neutralizing the pH value. This considerably improves the effect of the drugs administered in addition.

7.2 Actovegin®

Actovegin®, which I have been using for more than 40 years, is a physiologically balanced blend of hydrolyzed essential amino acids, obtained through microfiltration of calf blood, which we use to treat all muscle injuries.

The amino acids are incorporated into both the glycoplastic energy metabolism and the repair metabolism of the injured muscle fiber systems. According to the doping regulations of the World Anti-Doping Agency (WADA), there is no prohibition to use this preparation.

Only a few years ago, scientists from the Ludwig-Maximilians-University of Munich and the Sports University of Cologne asked themselves why I have been sticking with Actovegin® for decades despite all public criticism and have initiated a scientific study to investigate the effects of the preparation [5].

The result: It promotes the healing process of muscle injuries through a proven activation of the satellite cells on the muscle cell membranes so that the new formation of muscle fibers is stimulated and scarring from collagen fibers is avoided.

In addition, a further study (2020) demonstrated a suspected anti-inflammatory effect [10].

7.3 Vitamins A, C and E

In addition, in the case of structural muscle injuries, the capacity of free radical scavengers is improved locally and systemically by appropriate administration of the antioxidative vitamins A, C and E. As a result, the "free radicals" (highly reactive, very aggressive atoms, ions or molecules with an unpaired electron pair) released as a result of the injury are better intercepted and cell membrane damage is limited.

7.4 Zinc

Since the zinc level drops significantly during the acute phase reaction – and even more so in the event of injury – zinc is also substituted. Zinc ions are essential for the protein biosynthesis of amino acids. Zinc stabilizes the synthesis-promoting ribonucleic acid (RNA), acts as a free radical scavenger at the site of the injury and is involved in the phagocytosis of granulocytes. Zinc ions are applied intravenously and later per os to promote protein synthesis.

7.5   Magnesium

As we know, injuries cause a particularly high release of mineralocorticoids, resulting in an even more severe loss of electrolytes and trace elements than in the usual acute phase reaction in sports. For this reason, magnesium is additionally substituted, otherwise, the metabolism of the energy-rich muscle phosphates would be impaired.

7.6   Enzymes

As part of the post-traumatic reaction after muscle injuries, swelling and an inflammatory reaction occur locally in the tissue. In order to limit this reaction to a physiological level necessary for healing, the oral intake of fibrinolytic and anti-inflammatory enzymes (Wobenzym®, Phlogenzym®, Bromelain) is recommended. The partial fibrinolysis and proteolysis induced by these enzymes minimize the release of inflammatory and phagocytic mediators and consequently reduce the inflammatory phase, resulting in faster healing.

8 Critical evaluation of magnetic resonance imaging of muscle injuries

MRI (magnetic resonance imaging) is a valuable tool in the diagnosis of many injuries or degenerative changes, but not in muscular disorders. The occasionally very impressive images often lead – I mean in considerably more than 50% of cases – to misinterpretation, even misdiagnosis and usually to overinterpretation! Thus, after increasingly frequent use of MRI diagnostics, the number of muscle bundle tears has multiplied in recent years. For example, in a German soccer league club, there were more than 20 such diagnoses in one season! However, muscle bundle tears are rather rare and represent on average one or two such serious injuries per season per team. Instead, the clinical findings are crucial here!

It is mainly the neurogenic muscle hardenings that are often falsely diagnosed as muscle bundle tears. The fluid detected by the MRI is merely congested lymphatic fluid and not a hematoma, as usually assumed by radiologists. If the lymph stasis increases, it forces the muscle fibers out of the displayed layered planes. As a result, this may appear as a disruption in the muscle fibers, when it is not.

This leads to the diagnosis of torn muscle fibers, torn muscle bundles, torn fascia and tendon injuries, even though in reality there is no structural injury. As expected, the muscle and tendon fibers that were not injured or displaced over their entire length return to their original layered plane (smooth and without any tortuosity) after relieving the fluid accumulation.

In the case of a hematoma resulting from a tear injury, we see a similar displacement phenomenon, namely that the muscle fiber interruption appears to be greater than it actually is.

This means for the clinical practice:

The evaluation of MRI images is all too often dependent on the amount of fluid displayed. It makes no difference whether the fluid is edema, hematoma or injection fluid, whereby the structural damage interpreted into it is frequently not present at all. Incorrectly it is assumed, the more fluid is displayed, the greater the damage.

Functional injuries that do not lead to a rupture of muscle fibers, such as the muscle strain or neurogenic muscle hardening (the last-named more frequently) are not even mentioned in radiology.

In this review article we have intentionally refrained from showing MRI images. Even we, as sports orthopedists, who have been taking MRI images of athletes with muscle injuries for decades, do not consider ourselves capable of making an exact diagnosis solely on these images. Only by combining imaging, the history and clinical examination it is possible to establish an exact diagnosis and thus a correct treatment strategy. In our clinic, we have an excellent interdisciplinary cooperation between sports orthopedics and radiology.

8.1 Patient cases with incorrect diagnosis after magnetic resonance imaging

A concrete example of a misjudgment of a pulled muscle was found in a Premier League player after an MRI examination in England:

The player – a German national player – injured himself in the first half of an international match. After thorough diagnosis through palpation and functional tests in the halftime break and confirmed diagnosis, the first therapeutic measures (such as muscle release, strain-counterstrain as well as spray and stretch) were already initiated.

These applications had already brought about an improvement in symptoms. Afterward, our infiltration therapy was applied, an ointment bandage was applied and the player was treated with medication. The player's club was informed of the measures in writing.

The next day – after the player had returned to his home club – the club doctor arranged for an MRI scan. The diagnosis: torn muscle bundle. A pause of several weeks was scheduled. The infiltra-

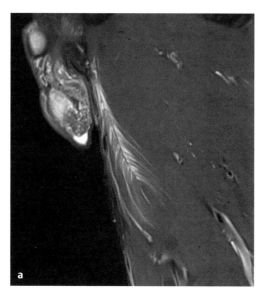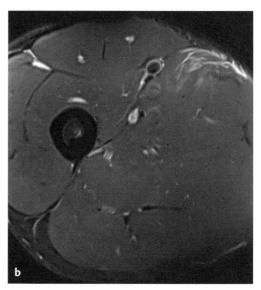

Fig. **11**   MRI imaging in sagittal (**a**) and axial (**b**) planes of neurogenic muscle hardening with long-distance lymphatic stasis in the left adductor musculature.

tion solution that was not yet metabolized and still visible was incorrectly considered a hematoma. However, the healing process progressed quickly, the player was able to train again after a few days and play a league match after nine days.

In the last few weeks, I have seen five externally incorrectly diagnosed muscle bundle tears of various Bundesliga players, in which not even a few fibers were torn. In each case it was a neurogenic muscle hardening. The associated lymphatic stasis is very characteristic of the injury and can be recognized by the pattern of distribution: long-distance intramuscular (inside the fascia) and possibly also long-distance and/or circumscribed intermuscular (outside the fascia) lymphatic stasis.

To illustrate the difficulty of interpreting solely MRI images for diagnosis, a magnetic resonance tomography of a player will be presented here as an exception (Fig. **11**). Here, an extensive and long-distance fluid infiltration in the area of the adductors is shown, suggesting a pronounced muscle injury. However, this is merely a pure lymphatic stasis in the region of the adductor longus muscle.

After treatment of the cause and lymphatic drainage, the player was able to resume running exercises two days later. The cause was simply a

neurogenic muscle hardening and not a structural muscle injury. We found the cause in the area of the left sacroiliac joint, which had caused irritation of the obturator nerve as a consequence of a blockage. As a result, an increase in muscle tone (adductor longus muscle) and a dysfunction in lymphatic drainage regulation (lymphatic congestion) developed in the supply area of this nerve.

Repeatedly, I have heard from athletes that the injury had not been clinically examined at all, but that they had been told: "*Go straight to MRI!*" Radiologists describe and evaluate images. They usually do not know the history of the athlete, the symptoms of the injury, or palpation findings. A major deficiency in sports medicine!

What does it mean for the player and the club if such an incorrect radiological diagnosis (torn muscle bundle) occurs? At least four weeks of unnecessary absence and an absolute loss of form of the player. The players mentioned above and treated by us were back in team training at the latest after two weeks and not, as is absolutely necessary with torn muscle bundles, after six weeks. Sport and match reports of the sports editorial offices prove this.

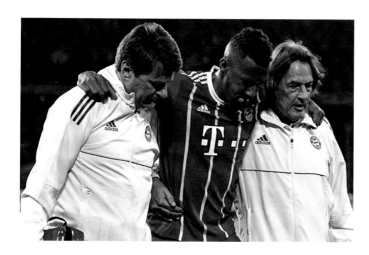

Fig. **12** Jérôme Boateng can only leave the field with support after a torn adductor muscle bundle (2018).

"How could we be responsible for questioning the MRI in such a way and ignoring it?" My answer: *"By carefully palpating and finding no muscle fiber disruption."* Furthermore, the MRI diagnosis did not correspond at all to the medical history and symptoms expressed by the players.

From over 40 years of experience in the medical care of top athletes, I can say: "In the case of such a severe and rather rare muscle injury (torn muscle bundle), the person affected reports a pain similar to a knife stab, falls to the ground and does not even try to get up again." Under no circumstances does he leave the court without help (Fig. **12**). Even in the case of a torn muscle fiber, he carefully limps and leaves the court or playing field. This was not the case with any of the injured players mentioned.

At this point I would also like to mention the MRI findings after a muscle contusion with a hematoma. Even if the images give the impression that there is a larger tissue rupture, it is merely a tissue contusion. The mechanism is not suitable to cause muscle fibers to tear and, as a rule, muscle fibers are not structurally damaged. After suitable therapy, soccer players, for example, can return to team training after a few days.

I, therefore, appeal to all sports physicians who increasingly rely on magnetic resonance imaging for the diagnosis of muscle injuries and thus take themselves out of the responsibility to train themselves in palpation, to refer to the relevant literature and to take the physiotherapists on board for the diagnosis. They are usually experienced experts

in their field. It is a wonderful opportunity to exchange ideas with them.

After all, I also recommend a better exchange between sports physicians and radiologists so that such misdiagnoses are avoided (practice-oriented versus theoretical medicine).

The commonly false findings are likely to confuse athletes, even if they can already train again without pain. It is not acceptable that a radiologist misinterprets a lymphatic stasis or a lymphatic drainage disorder that persists for weeks after the injury – caused by adhesions, scar distortions or even a neurogenic etiology – and declares that the injury has not healed.

It is unacceptable that radiologists – generally no sports physicians – use their MRI images to make muscle injury diagnoses and even make rehabilitation recommendations.

Nor is it acceptable that empirical knowledge accumulated over 40 years in high-performance sports should be turned upside down. We keep treating patients, not images.

We, as sports physicians, are overloaded with statistical surveys and results of large-scale muscle injury studies. In my opinion, many of them are misleading, since often the diagnoses (MRI-based) are wrong. As a result, published studies must be assessed very critically in some cases. For example, even in the very extensive and meaningful studies by Ekstrand et al., the quality of the evaluation depends on the diagnosis of the respective team physicians of the soccer teams. In my opinion, the severity of muscle injuries is sometimes overinterpreted in these studies [9, 10].

My hope for the further development of MRI technology is that MRI images will in the future make it possible to distinguish between lymph stasis and hematoma on the day of the injury and that MRI technology will be significantly improved.

This would mean a major advance in the diagnosis of muscle injuries.

For more detailed information I would like to refer to my textbook "Muscle Injuries in Sports" (Thieme Publishers) [11].

References

1 Mueller-Wohlfahrt H-W, Haensel L, Mithoefer K et al. Terminology and classification of muscle injuries in sport: The Munich consensus statement. Br J Sports Med 2013; 47: 342–350. doi:10.1136/bjsports-2012-091448

2 Dimmick S, Linklater JM. Imaging of Acute Hamstring Muscle Strain Injuries. Semin Musculoskelet Radiol 2017; 21: 415–432. doi:10.1055/s-0037-1604005

3 Pollock N, James S, Lee J et al. British athletics muscle injury classification: A new grading system. Br J Sports Med 2014; 48: 1347–1351. doi:10.1136/bjsports-2013-093302

4 Dimitriou M. Human muscle spindle sensitivity reflects the balance of activity between antagonistic muscles. J Neurosci 2014; 34: 13644–13655. doi:10.1523/jneurosci.2611-14.2014

5 Reichl FX, Holdt LM, Teupser D et al. Comprehensive Analytics of Actovegin® and Its Effect on Muscle Cells. Int J Sports Med 2017; 38: 809–818. doi:10.1055/s-0043-115738

6 Porozov S, Cahalon L, Weiser M et al. Inhibition of IL-1beta and TNF-alpha secretion from resting and activated human immunocytes by the homeopathic medication Traumeel S. Clin Dev Immunol 2004; 11: 143–149. doi:10.1080/10446670410001722203

7 St Laurent G 3rd, Seilheimer B, Tackett M et al. Deep Sequencing Transcriptome Analysis of Murine Wound Healing: Effects of a Multicomponent, Multitarget Natural Product Therapy-Tr14. Front Mol Biosci 2017; 4: 57. doi:10.3389/fmolb.2017.00057

8 Reichl FX, Högg C, Liu F et al. Actovegin® reduces PMA-induced inflammation on human cells. Eur J Appl Physiol 2020; 120: 1671–1680. doi:10.1007/s00421-020-04398-2

9 Ekstrand J, Hägglund M, Waldén M. Injury incidence and injury patterns in professional football: the UEFA injury study. Br J Sports Med 2011; 45: 553–558. doi:10.1136/bjsm.2009.060582

10 Ekstrand J, Hägglund M, Waldén M. Epidemiology of muscle injuries in professional football (soccer). Am J Sports Med 2011; 39: 1226–1232. doi:10.1177/0363546510395879

11 Müller-Wohlfahrt H-W, Uebelacker P, Garrett WE jr, Hänsel L. Muscle Injuries in Sports. Stuttgart: Thieme; 2013